Keto Diet Cookbook

The best beginner's guide recipes of other keto favorite quick and easy for lose your weight
Book 1

Sophie Toy

© Copyright 2021 All rights reserved.

The following Book is reproduced below with the goal of providing information that is as accurate and reliable as possible. Regardless, purchasing this Book can be seen as consent to the fact that both the publisher and the author of this book are in no way experts on the topics discussed within and that any recommendations or suggestions that are made herein are for entertainment purposes only. Professionals should be consulted as needed prior to undertaking any of the action endorsed herein.

This declaration is deemed fair and valid by both the American Bar Association and the Committee of Publishers Association and is legally binding throughout the United States.

Furthermore, the transmission, duplication, or reproduction of any of the following work including specific information will be considered an illegal act irrespective of if it is done electronically or in print. This extends to creating a secondary or tertiary copy of the work or a recorded copy and is only allowed with the express written consent from the Publisher. All additional right reserved.

The information in the following pages is broadly considered a truthful and accurate account of facts and as such, any inattention, use, or misuse of the information in question by the reader will render any resulting actions solely under their purview. There are no scenarios in which the publisher or the original author of this work can be in any fashion deemed liable for any hardship or damages that may befall them after undertaking information described herein.

Additionally, the information in the following pages is intended only for informational purposes and should thus be thought of as universal. As befitting its nature, it is presented without assurance regarding its prolonged validity or interim quality. Trademarks that are mentioned are done without written consent and can in no way be considered an endorsement from the trademark holder.

Table of Contents

1. BROCCOLI CHEESE SOUP 1
2. CHIPOTLE PIZZA WITH COTIJA & CILANTRO 3
3. RASPBERRY & RUM OMELET 5
4. CHEESY HERB OMELET 7
5. BACON LOADED EGGPLANTS 9
6. VANILLA-COCONUT CREAM TART 11
7. EGG & CHEESE STUFFED PEPPERS 13
8. CARROT & CHEESE MOUSSE 15
9. CRABMEAT & CHEESE STUFFED AVOCADO 17
10. CHEESE, HAM AND EGG MUFFINS 19
11. PROSCIUTTO & CHEESE EGG CUPS 21
12. CHORIZO EGG BALLS 23
13. HERBED KETO BREAD 25
14. QUATRO FORMAGGIO PIZZA 27
15. MINI EGG MUFFINS 29
16. GRILLED HALLOUMI CHEESE WITH EGGS 31
17. CREAMY CHEDDAR DEVILED EGGS 33
18. ITALIAN-STYLE EGG MUFFINS 35
19. CLASSIC SPICY EGG SALAD 37
20. ASIAGO, PEPPERONI, AND PEPPER CASSEROLE 39
21. FESTIVE ZUCCHINI BOATS 41
22. NANA'S PICKLED EGGS 43
23. MUSHROOM AND CHEESE WRAPS 45
24. EGG DROP SOUP WITH TOFU 47
25. CAULIFLOWER "MAC" AND CHEESE CASSEROLE 49
26. BAKED CHEESE-STUFFED TOMATOES 51

27 . SPICY CHEESE OMELET WITH CHERVIL	53
28 . SCRAMBLED EGGS WITH CRABMEAT	55
29 . BLUE CHEESE AND SOPPRESSATA BALLS	57
30 . ALFREDO CHEESE DIP	59
31 . GENOVESE SALAMI AND EGG FAT BOMBS	61
32 . ASPARAGUS & TARRAGON FLAN	63
33 . TOFU SANDWICH WITH CABBAGE SLAW	65
34 . LEMON CAULIFLOWER "COUSCOUS" WITH HALLOUMI	67
35 . ZUCCHINI LASAGNA WITH RICOTTA & SPINACH	69
36 . CREAMY VEGETABLE STEW	71
37 . SALAMI & PRAWN PIZZA	73
38 . PORK & VEGETABLE TART	75
39 . HAM & EGG SALAD	77
40 . GREEK YOGURT & CHEESE ALFREDO SAUCE	79
41 . BROCCOLI RABE PIZZA WITH PARMESAN	81
42 . CHORIZO SCOTCH EGGS	83
43 . MEDITERRANEAN CHEESE BALLS	85
44 . HAM & EGG MUG CUPS	87
45 . CAULIFLOWER & GOUDA CHEESE CASSEROLE	89
46 . CREMINI MUSHROOM STROGANOFF	91
47 . SRIRACHA TOFU WITH YOGURT SAUCE	93
48 . WILD MUSHROOM & ASPARAGUS STEW	95
49 . KETO PIZZA MARGHERITA	97
50 . CAULIFLOWER RISOTTO WITH MUSHROOMS	99
51 . WALNUT TOFU SAUTÉ	101
52 . SPAGHETTI SQUASH WITH EGGPLANT & PARMESAN	103
53 . FRIED TOFU WITH MUSHROOMS	105
54 . VEGETABLE TEMPURA	107
55 . SPANISH-STYLE SAUSAGE AND EGGS	109

56 . KETO BELGIAN WAFFLES 111
57 . SCOTCH EGGS WITH GROUND PORK.. 113

1. Broccoli Cheese Soup

INGREDIENTS (4 servings)

2 tbsp butter ½ cup leeks, chopped 1 celery stalk, chopped 1 serrano pepper, finely chopped 1 tsp garlic puree ½ lb broccoli florets 3 cups chicken stock 1 cup coconut milk 1 tsp mustard powder 6 oz Monterey Jack cheese, grated Salt and black pepper to taste 2 tbsp fresh parsley, chopped

DIRECTIONS (20 minutes)

Set a pot over medium heat and melt butter. Add in serrano pepper, celery, and leeks and sauté for 5 minutes until soft. Stir in garlic puree and mustard powder for 1 minute. Pour in chicken stock and coconut milk. Bring to a Boil and reduce the heat. Allow simmering for 10 minutes. Add in the broccoli. Cook for another 5 minutes. Remove from the heat and fold in the cheese. Stir to ensure the cheese is melted, and you have a homogenous mixture. Adjust the seasoning, top with parsley, and serve warm.

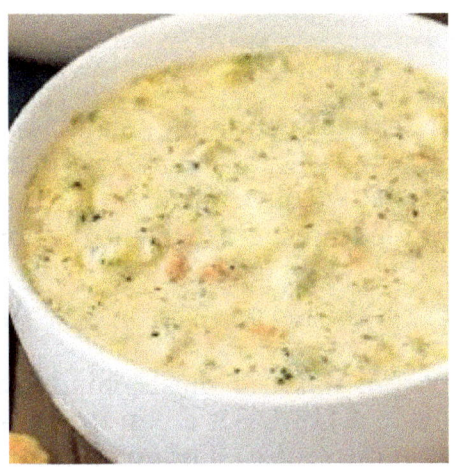

Notes:

2. Chipotle Pizza with Cotija & Cilantro

INGREDIENTS (2 servings)

Pizza crust 4 eggs, beaten ¼ cup sour cream 2 tbsp flaxseed meal 1 tsp chipotle pepper ¼ tsp cumin ½ tsp dried ground coriander ¼ tsp salt 1 tbsp olive oil 2 tbsp tomato paste 2 oz Cotija cheese, shredded 1 tbsp fresh cilantro, chopped

DIRECTIONS (15 minutes)

Mix eggs, sour cream, flaxseed meal, chipotle pepper, cumin, coriander, and salt in a bowl. Set a pan over medium heat and warm ½ tablespoon oil. Ladle ½ of crust mixture into the pan and evenly spread out. Cook until the edges are set, flip, and cook on the second side. Repeat with the remaining crust mixture. Warm the remaining ½ tablespoon of oil in the pan. Spread each pizza crust with tomato paste, then scatter over the cotija cheese. In batches, bake in the oven for 8-10 minutes at 425°F until all the cheese melts. Garnish with cilantro and serve.

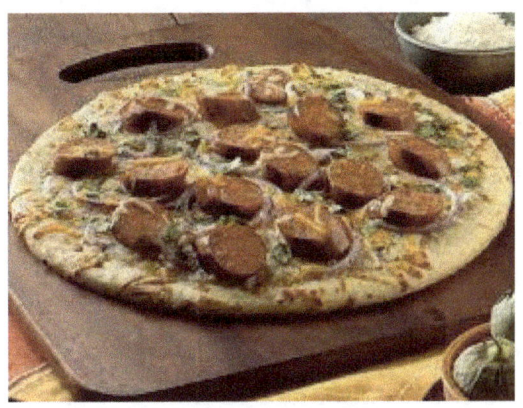

Notes:

3. Raspberry & Rum Omelet

INGREDIENTS (1 servings)

2 eggs 2 tbsp heavy cream ½ tsp ground cloves 1 tbsp coconut oil 2 tbsp mascarpone cheese 6 fresh raspberries, sliced ½ tsp powdered swerve sugar 1 tbsp rum

DIRECTIONS (10 minutes)

Beat the eggs with ground cloves and heavy cream. Set pan over medium heat and warm oil. Place in the egg mixture and cook for 3 minutes. Set the omelet onto a plate. Top with raspberries and mascarpone cheese. Roll it up and sprinkle with powdered swerve. Pour the warm rum over the omelet and ignite it. Let the flame die out and serve.

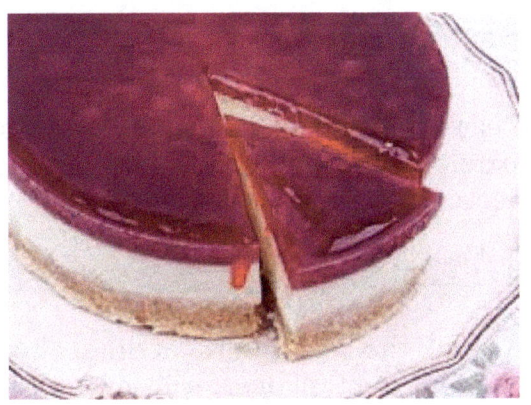

Notes:

4. Cheesy Herb Omelet

INGREDIENTS (2 servings)

4 slices cooked bacon, crumbled 4 eggs, beaten 1 tsp basil, chopped 1 tsp parsley, chopped Salt and black pepper to taste ½ cup cheddar cheese, grated

DIRECTIONS (10 minutes)

In a frying pan, cook the bacon until sizzling, about 5 minutes. Add in eggs, parsley, black pepper, salt, and basil. Scatter the cheese over half of the omelet and, using a spatula, fold in half over the filling. Cook for 1 extra minute or until cooked through and serve immediately.

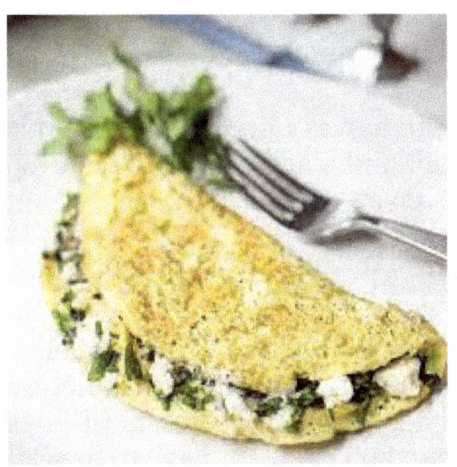

Notes:

5. Bacon Loaded Eggplants

INGREDIENTS (4 servings)

2 eggplants, cut into halves 1 onion, chopped 4 bacon slices, chopped 4 eggs Salt and black pepper to taste ¼ tsp dried parsley Preheat oven at 380°F.

DIRECTIONS (35 minutes)

Scoop flesh from eggplant halves to make shells. Set the eggplant boats on a greased baking pan. Heat a skillet over medium heat and stir-fry the bacon for 5 minutes until crispy. Remove to a plate. Add the onion and eggplant flesh to the skillet and sauté for 5-7 minutes until tender. Season with salt, pepper, and parsley and stir in the bacon. Divide the mixture between the eggplant shells. Crack an egg in each half, sprinkle with salt and pepper, and bake for 30 minutes or until the boats become tender and the eggs are set. Serve with tomato salad.

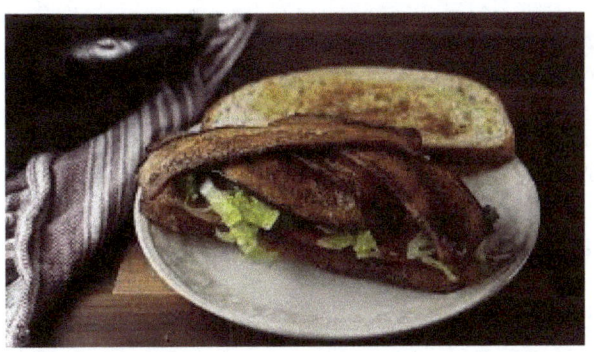

Notes:

6. Vanilla-Coconut Cream Tart

INGREDIENTS (6 servings)

½ cup butter ⅓ cup xylitol ¾ cup coconut flour ⅓ cup coconut shreds, unsweetened 2 ¼ cups heavy cream 3 egg yolks ⅓ cup almond flour ¾ cup water ½ tsp ground cinnamon ½ tsp star anise, ground ½ tsp vanilla extract 2 tbsp coconut flakes

DIRECTIONS (30 minutes)

Warm butter in a pan over medium heat. Stir in xylitol and cook until fully dissolved. Add in coconut shreds and coconut flour and cook for 2 minutes. Scrape the crust mixture into a baking dish. Refrigerate. In the same pan, warm 1 ¼ cups of heavy cream over medium heat. Fold in egg yolks and mix thoroughly. Mix in water and almond flour until thick. Place in cinnamon, vanilla, and anise star. Cook until thick. Let cool for 10 minutes; sprinkle over the crust. Place in the fridge for 2 hours. Beat the remaining heavy cream until stiff peaks start to form. Spread the cream all over the cake. Top with coconut flakes to serve.

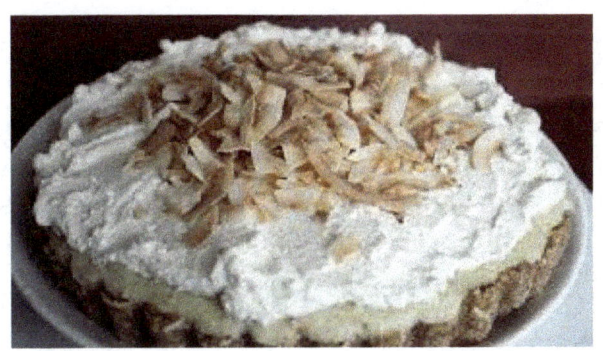

Notes:

7. Egg & Cheese Stuffed Peppers

INGREDIENTS (4 servings)

4 bell peppers, tops sliced off and deseeded 6 oz cottage cheese, crumbled 6 oz blue cheese, crumbled ½ cup pork rinds, crushed 2 cloves garlic, smashed 1 ½ cups pureed tomatoes 1 tsp dried basil 1 tbsp olive oil ½ tsp chili pepper 2 eggs, beaten Preheat oven to 360°F.

DIRECTIONS (35 minutes)

In a bowl, mix garlic, cottage cheese, pork rinds, blue cheese, eggs, tomatoes, chili pepper, and basil. Stuff the peppers and place them in a greased casserole dish. Pour in 1 cup of water. Drizzle with olive oil. Bake for 30 minutes until the peppers are tender. Serve with mixed salad.

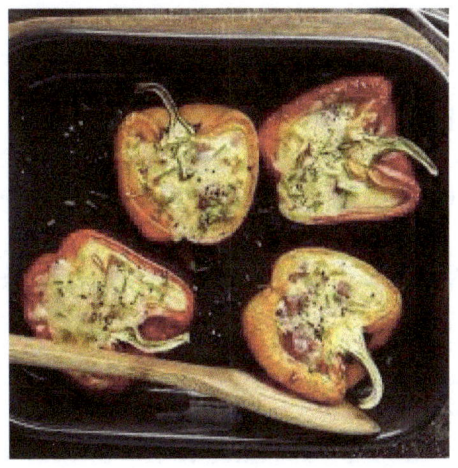

Notes:

8. Carrot & Cheese Mousse

INGREDIENTS (6 servings)

1 ½ cups half & half ½ cup cream cheese, softened ½ cup erythritol 3 eggs 1 ¼ cups canned carrots ½ tsp ground cloves ½ tsp ground cinnamon ¼ tsp grated nutmeg A pinch of salt

DIRECTIONS (15 minutes)

Heat a pan over medium heat, mix erythritol, cream cheese, and half & half and warm, stirring frequently. Remove from the heat. Beat the eggs; slowly place in ½ of the hot cream mixture to the beaten eggs. Pour the mixture back to the pan. Cook for 3 minutes, until thick. Kill the heat; add in carrots, cinnamon, salt, nutmeg, and cloves. Blend with a blender. Let cool before serving.

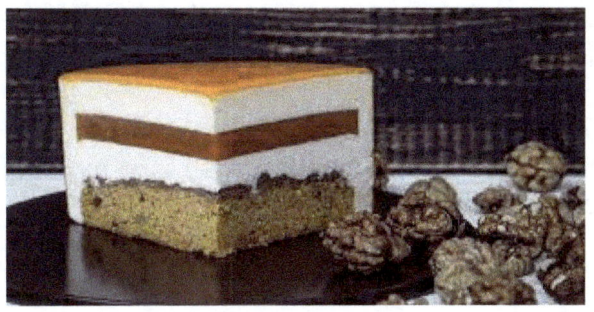

Notes:

9. Crabmeat & Cheese Stuffed Avocado

INGREDIENTS (4 servings)

1 tsp olive oil 1 cup crabmeat 2 avocados, halved and pitted 3 oz cream cheese ¼ cup almonds, chopped 1 tsp smoked paprika Preheat oven to 425°F.

DIRECTIONS (25 minutes)

In a bowl, mix crabmeat with cream cheese. Fill the avocado halves with crabmeat mixture and top with almonds. Bake for 18 minutes. Decorate with smoked paprika and serve.

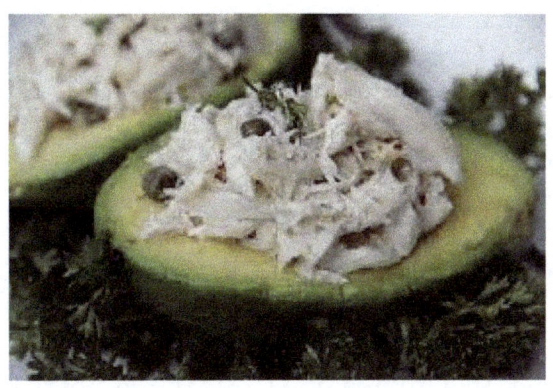

Notes:

10. Cheese, Ham and Egg Muffins

INGREDIENTS (6 servings)

24 slices smoked ham 6 eggs, beaten Salt and black pepper to taste ¼ cup fresh parsley, chopped ¼ cup ricotta cheese ¼ cup Brie, chopped Preheat oven to 390°F.

DIRECTIONS (20 minutes)

Line 2 slices of smoked ham into each greased muffin cup, to circle each mold. In a mixing bowl, mix the rest of the ingredients. Fill ¾ of the ham lined muffin cup with the egg/cheese mixture. Bake for 15 minutes. Serve warm!

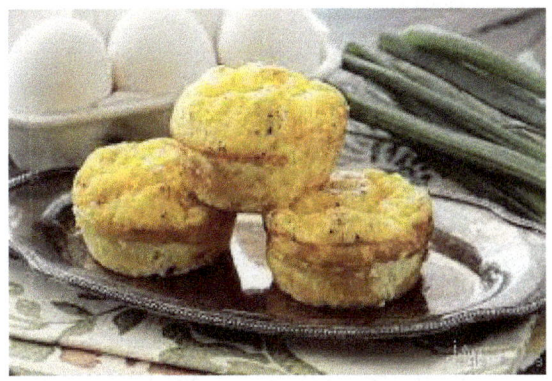

Notes:

11. Prosciutto & Cheese Egg Cups

INGREDIENTS (4 servings)

4 slices prosciutto 4 eggs 2 green onions, chopped ½ cup cheddar cheese, shredded ¼ tsp garlic powder Salt and black pepper to taste Preheat oven to 390°F.

DIRECTIONS (30 minutes)

Line the prosciutto slices on greased ramekins. In a bowl, combine the remaining ingredients. Split the egg mixture among the cups. Bake for 20 minutes. Leave to cool before serving.

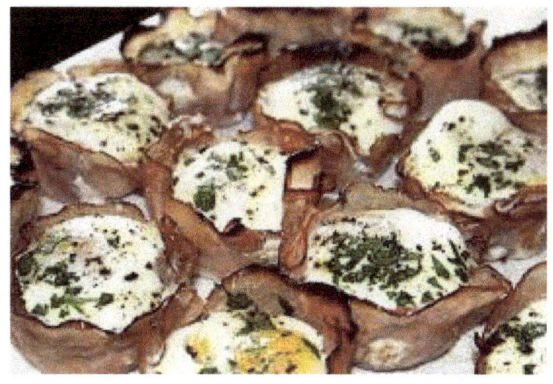

Notes:

12. Chorizo Egg Balls

INGREDIENTS (6 servings)

2 eggs ½ cup butter, softened 8 black olives, pitted and chopped 3 tbsp mayonnaise Salt to taste ½ tsp crushed red pepper flakes 1 lb cooked chorizo, chopped 2 tbsp chia seeds

DIRECTIONS (10 minutes)

In a food processor, place the eggs, olives, pepper flakes, mayo, butter, and salt and blitz until everything is incorporated. Stir in the chorizo. Refrigerate for 30 minutes. Form balls from the mixture. Roll the balls through the chia seeds to coat. Keep in the refrigerator until serving time.

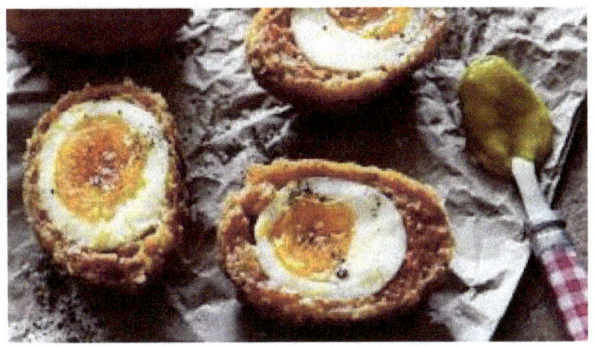

Notes:

13. Herbed Keto Bread

INGREDIENTS (6 servings)

5 eggs ½ tsp tartar cream 2 cups almond flour 3 tablespoons butter, melted 3 tsp baking powder 1 tsp salt ½ tsp dried oregano 1 tbsp sunflower seeds 2 tbsp sesame seeds Preheat oven to 360°F.

DIRECTIONS (40 minutes)

Combine the eggs with cream of tartar until the formation of stiff peaks happens. In a food processor, place in the baking powder, flour, salt, and butter and blitz to incorporate fully. Stir in the egg mixture. Scoop the batter into a greased loaf pan. Spread the loaf with sesame seeds, sunflower seeds, and oregano and bake for 35 minutes. Serve with butter.

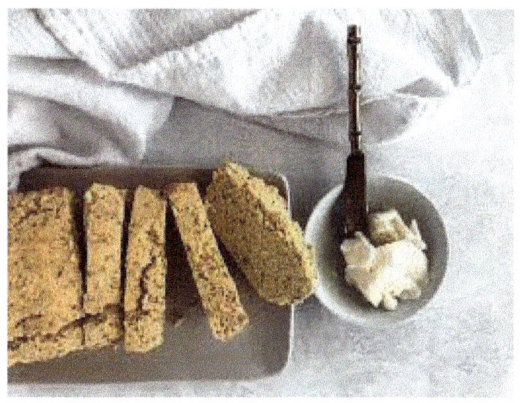

Notes:

14. Quatro Formaggio Pizza

INGREDIENTS (4 servings)

1 tbsp olive oil ½ cup cheddar cheese, shredded 1 ¼ cups mozzarella cheese, grated ½ cup mascarpone cheese ½ cup blue cheese 2 tbsp sour cream 2 garlic cloves, chopped 1 red bell pepper, sliced 1 green bell pepper, sliced 10 cherry tomatoes, halved 1 tsp oregano Salt and black pepper to taste

DIRECTIONS (15 minutes)

In a bowl, mix the cheeses. Set a pan over medium heat and warm olive oil. Spread the cheese mixture on the pan and cook for 5 minutes until cooked through. Scatter garlic and sour cream over the crust. Add in tomatoes and bell peppers; cook for 2 minutes. Sprinkle with pepper, salt, and oregano and serve.

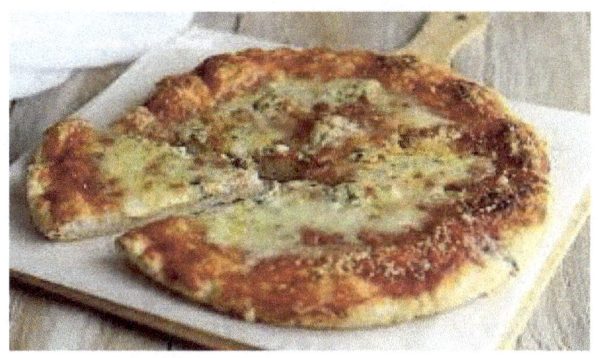

Notes:

15. Mini Egg Muffins

INGREDIENTS (6 servings)

2 tbsp olive oil 1 onion, chopped 1 bell pepper, chopped 6 slices bacon, chopped 6 eggs, whisked 1 cup gruyere cheese, shredded Salt and black pepper to taste ¼ tsp rosemary 1 tbsp fresh parsley, chopped Preheat oven to 390°F.

DIRECTIONS (40 minutes)

Place cupcake liners to your muffin pan. In a skillet over medium heat, warm the olive oil and sauté the onion and bell pepper for 4-5 minutes as you stir constantly until tender. Stir in bacon and cook for 3 more minutes. Add in the rest of the ingredients and mix well. Set the mixture to the lined muffin pan and bake for 23 minutes. Let muffins cool before serving.

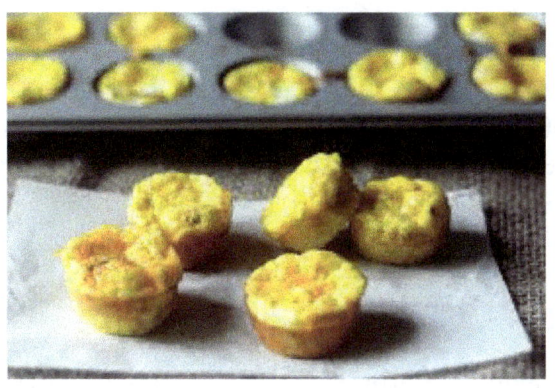

Notes:

16. Grilled Halloumi Cheese with Eggs

INGREDIENTS (4 servings)

4 slices halloumi cheese 2 tbsp olive oil 1 tsp dried Greek seasoning blend 6 eggs, beaten ½ tsp sea salt ¼ tsp crushed red pepper flakes 1 ½ cups avocado, pitted and sliced 1 cup grape tomatoes, halved 4 tbsp pecans, chopped

DIRECTIONS (20 minutes)

Preheat your grill to medium. Set the halloumi in the center of a piece of heavy-duty foil. Sprinkle oil over the halloumi and apply Greek seasoning blend. Close the foil to create a packet. Grill for about 15 minutes. Then slice into four pieces. In a frying pan over medium heat, warm the olive oil and cook the eggs. Stir well to create large and soft curds. Season with salt and red pepper flakes. Put the eggs and grilled cheese on a serving bowl. Serve alongside tomatoes and avocado, decorated with chopped pecans.

Notes:

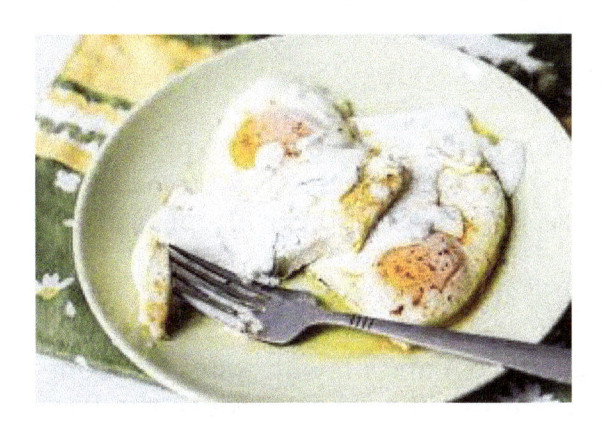

17. Creamy Cheddar Deviled Eggs

INGREDIENTS (4 servings)

8 eggs ¼ cup mayonnaise 1 tbsp tomato paste 2 tbsp celery, chopped 2 tbsp carrot, chopped 2 tbsp chives, minced 2 tbsp cheddar cheese, grated Salt and black pepper to taste

DIRECTIONS (20 minutes)

Place the eggs in a pot and fill with water by about 1 inch. Bring the eggs to a boil over high heat, reduce the heat to medium; simmer for 10 minutes. Remove and rinse under running water until cooled. Peel and discard the shell. Slice each egg in half lengthwise and get rid of the yolks. Mix the yolks with the rest of the ingredients. Split the mixture amongst the egg whites and set deviled eggs on a plate to serve.

Notes:

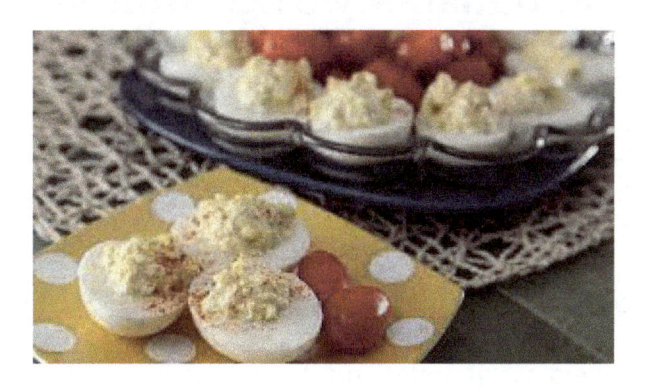

18. Italian-Style Egg Muffins

INGREDIENTS (3 servings)

6 eggs 1 pound beef sausages, chopped 1 tablespoon olive oil 1 cup Romano cheese, freshly grated Sea salt and black pepper, to season 1/2 teaspoon cayenne pepper

DIRECTIONS (10 minutes)

Whisk the eggs until pale and frothy. Add in the remaining ingredients and stir to combine. Pour the mixture into a lightly greased muffin pan. Bake in the preheated oven at 400 degrees F for 5 to 6 minutes.Bon appétit!

Notes:

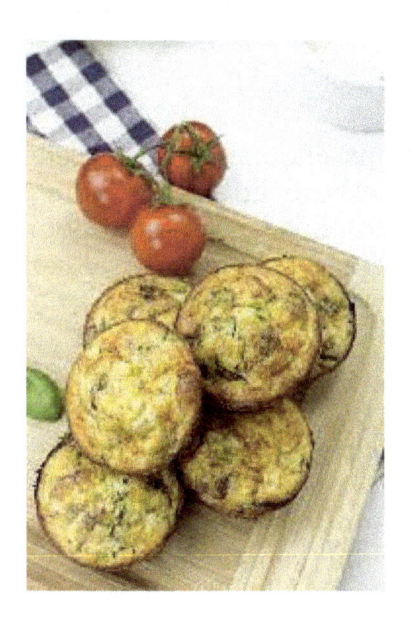

19. Classic Spicy Egg Salad

INGREDIENTS (8 servings)

10 eggs 1/2 cup onions, chopped 1/2 cup celery with leaves, chopped 2 cups butterhead lettuce, torn into pieces 3/4 cup mayonnaise 1 teaspoon hot sauce 1 tablespoon Dijon mustard 1/2 teaspoon fresh lemon juice Kosher salt and black pepper, to taste

DIRECTIONS (15 minutes)

Place the eggs in a saucepan and cover them with water by 1 inch. Cover and bring the water to a boil over high heat. Boil for 6 to 7 minutes over medium-high heat. Peel the eggs and chop them coarsely. Add in the remaining ingredients and toss to combine.Bon appétit!

Notes:

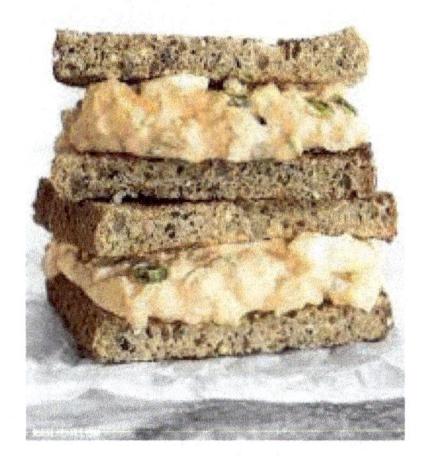

20. Asiago, Pepperoni, and Pepper Casserole

INGREDIENTS (4 servings)

8 eggs Salt and pepper, to taste 1 cup Asiago cheese, grated 1/2 cup cream cheese 1 bell pepper, chopped 1 chili pepper, deveined and chopped 1 teaspoon yellow mustard 8 slices pepperoni, chopped

DIRECTIONS (35 minutes)

In a mixing bowl, combine the eggs, salt, pepper, and cheese; spoon the mixture into a lightly greased baking dish. Add in the other ingredients. Bake in the preheated oven at 365 degrees F for about 30 minutes or until cooked through. Bon appétit!

Notes:

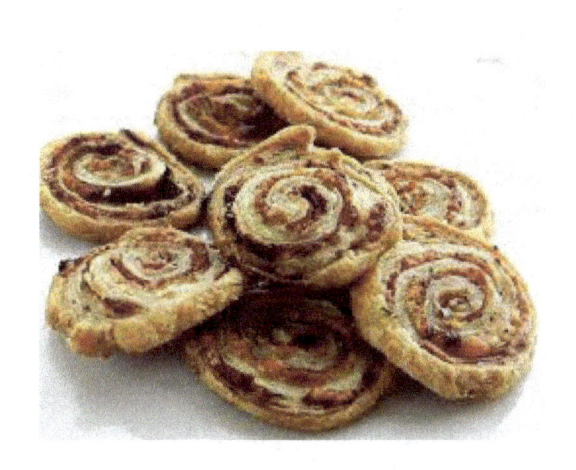

21. Festive Zucchini Boats

INGREDIENTS (3 servings)

3 medium-sized zucchinis, cut into halves and scoop out the pulp 6 eggs 1 tablespoon Dijon mustard 2 sausages, cooked and crumbled Salt and pepper, to taste 1/2 teaspoon dried basil

DIRECTIONS (35 minutes)

Place the zucchini boats on a lightly oiled baking sheet. Mix the Dijon mustard, sausages, salt, pepper, and basil. Spoon the sausage mixture into the zucchini shells. Crack an egg in each zucchini shell. Bake in the preheated oven at 390 degrees F for 30 to 35 minutes or until tender and cooked through.Enjoy!

Notes:

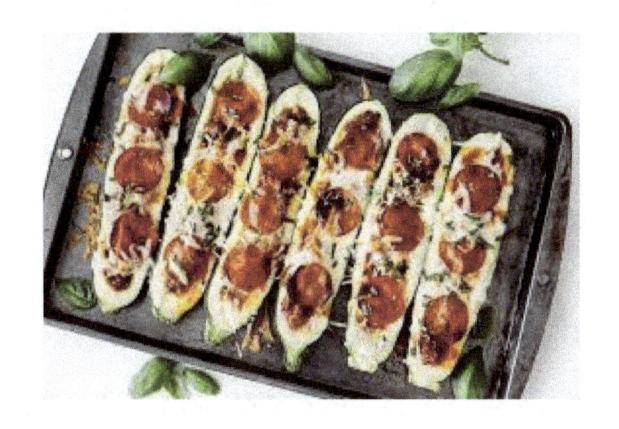

22. Nana's Pickled Eggs

INGREDIENTS (5 servings)

2 clove garlic, sliced 1 cup white vinegar 10 eggs 1 tablespoon yellow curry powder 1/2 cup onions, sliced 1 teaspoon fennel seeds 1 teaspoon mustard seeds 1 tablespoon sea salt 1 ¼ cups water

DIRECTIONS (20 minutes)

Place the eggs in a saucepan and cover them with water by 1 inch. Cover and bring the water to a boil over high heat. Boil for 6 to 7 minutes over medium-high heat. Peel the eggs and add them to a large-sized jar. Cook the other ingredients in a saucepan pan over moderately-high heat; bring to a boil. Immediately turn the heat to medium-low and continue to simmer for 5 to 6 minutes. Pour the mixture into the prepared jar.Bon appétit!

Notes:

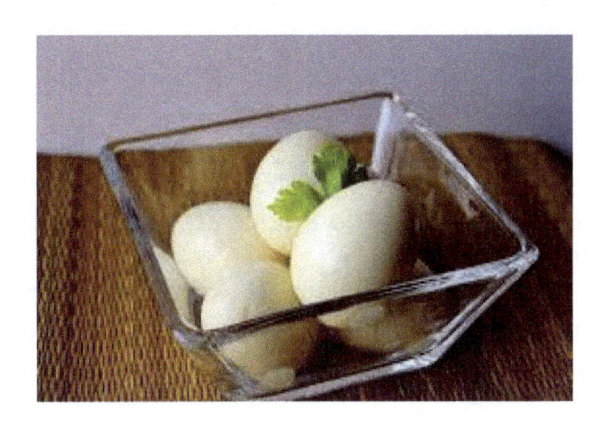

23. Mushroom and Cheese Wraps

INGREDIENTS (4 servings)

For the Wraps:
2 tablespoons cream cheese 6 eggs, separated into yolks and whites 1 tablespoon butter, room temperature Sea salt, to taste
For the Filling:
1 cup Cremini mushrooms, chopped 4 slices of Swiss cheese Salt and pepper, to taste 6-8 fresh arugula 1 teaspoon olive oil 1 large vine-ripened tomatoes, chopped

DIRECTIONS (20 minutes)

Mix all ingredients for the wraps until well combined. Prepare four wraps in a frying pan and set them aside. Next, heat 1 teaspoon of olive oil over a moderate heat. Cook the mushrooms until they release the liquid; season with salt and pepper.

Notes:

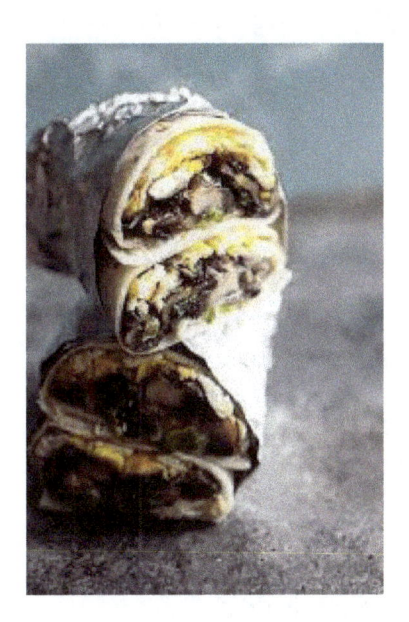

24. Egg Drop Soup with Tofu

INGREDIENTS (3 servings)

2 eggs, beaten 1/2 teaspoon curry paste 1/2 pound extra-firm tofu, cubed 2 cups vegetable broth 1 tablespoon coconut aminos 1 teaspoon butter, softened 1/4 teaspoon cayenne pepper Salt and ground black ground, to taste

DIRECTIONS (15 minutes)

In a heavy-bottomed pot, cook the broth, coconut aminos and butter over high heat; bring to a boil. Immediately turn the heat to a simmer. Stir in the eggs and curry paste, whisking constantly, until well incorporated. Add in the salt, black pepper, cayenne pepper, and tofu. Partially cover and continue to simmer approximately 2 minutes.Enjoy!

Notes:

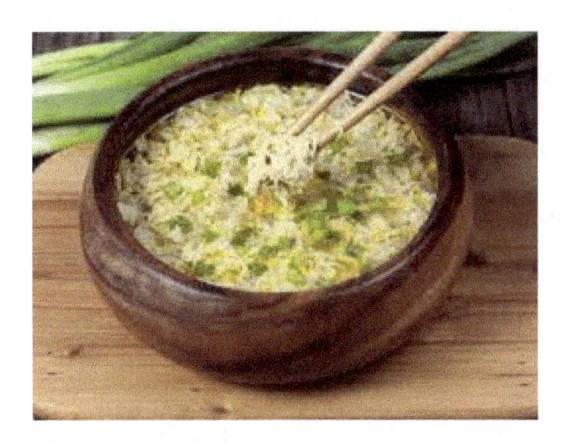

25. Cauliflower "Mac" and Cheese Casserole

INGREDIENTS (4 servings)

1 large-sized head cauliflower, broken into florets 1 cup Cottage cheese 1/2 cup milk 1/2 cup double cream 2 tablespoons olive oil 1 teaspoon garlic powder 1/2 teaspoon shallot powder 1 teaspoon dried parsley flakes Salt and pepper, to taste

DIRECTIONS (15 minutes)

Start by preheating your oven to 420 degrees F. In a lightly oiled baking dish, toss the cauliflower florets with the olive oil, salt, and pepper. Bake in the preheated oven for about 15 minutes. In a mixing dish, whisk the milk, cream, cheese, and spices. Pour the mixture over the cauliflower layer in the baking dish. Bake for another 10 minutes, until the top is hot and bubbly.Bon appétit!

Notes:

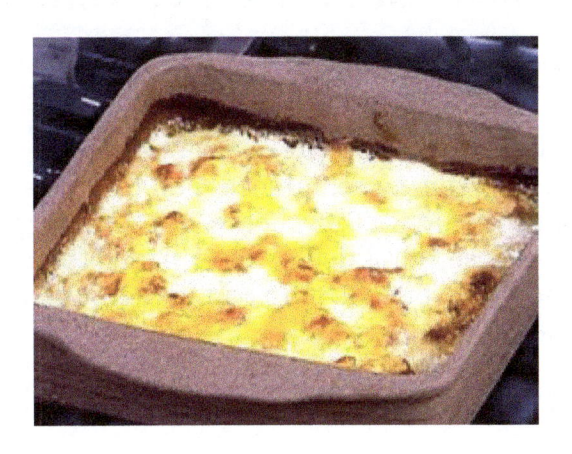

26. Baked Cheese-Stuffed Tomatoes

INGREDIENTS (5 servings)

2 teaspoons olive oil 1/4 cup Greek-style yogurt 1 egg, whisked 1 tablespoon fresh green garlic, minced 4 tablespoons fresh shallots, chopped 1 cup Ricotta cheese, at room temperature 1 ½ cups Swiss cheese, shredded 5 vine-ripened tomatoes, cut into halves and scoop out the pulp Salt and ground black pepper, to taste

DIRECTIONS (45 minutes)

Start by preheating your oven to 355 degrees F. Then, thoroughly combine the cheese, yogurt, egg, green garlic, shallots, salt, and pepper. Stuff the tomato halves with this filling. Brush the stuffed tomatoes with olive oil. Bake in the preheated oven for about 30 minutes.

Notes:

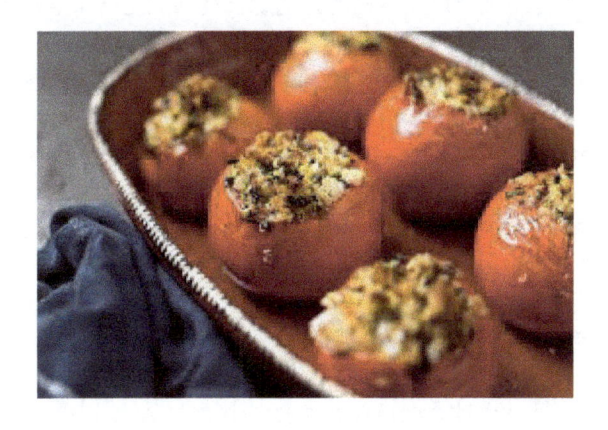

27. Spicy Cheese Omelet with Chervil

INGREDIENTS (2 servings)

4 eggs, beaten 1/2 cup Cheddar cheese, grated 2 tablespoons olive oil 1/2 teaspoon habanero pepper, minced 1/2 cup queso fresco cheese, crumbled 2 tablespoons fresh chervil, roughly chopped Salt and pepper, to taste

DIRECTIONS (15 minutes)

In a frying pan, heat the oil over a moderately high heat. Cook the eggs until the edges barely start setting. Add in the salt, pepper, habanero pepper, and cheese and cook an additional 4 minutes. Serve with fresh chervil. Bon appétit!

Notes:

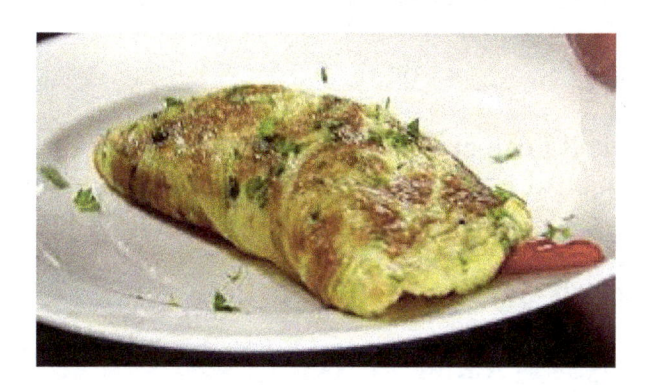

28. Scrambled Eggs with Crabmeat

INGREDIENTS (3 servings)

6 eggs, whisked 1 can crabmeat, flaked 1/2 teaspoon rosemary 1/2 teaspoon basil 1 tablespoon butter, room temperature For the Sauce: 1/2 teaspoon garlic, minced 3/4 cup cream cheese 1/2 cup onions, white and green parts, chopped 3 tablespoons mayonnaise Salt and black pepper, to taste

DIRECTIONS (15 minutes)

In a frying pan, melt the butter over a moderately high flame. Cook the eggs, gently stirring to create large soft curds. Cook until the eggs are barely set. Add in the crabmeat, rosemary and basil, and continue to cook, stirring frequently, until cooked through. Salt to taste. Make the sauce by whisking all ingredients.

Notes:

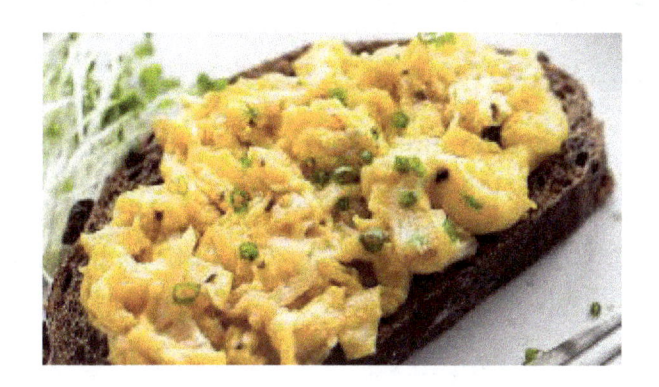

29. Blue Cheese and Soppressata Balls

INGREDIENTS (8 servings)

6 slices Soppressata, chopped 6 ounces Parmigiano-Reggiano cheese, grated 1 teaspoon baking powder 1 teaspoon garlic, minced 1 egg, whisked 1/2 teaspoon dried basil 1/2 teaspoon dried oregano 6 ounces cream cheese Salt and pepper, to taste 1/4 cup almond meal

DIRECTIONS (15 minutes)

Thoroughly combine all ingredients until well combined. Roll the mixture into bite-sized balls and arrange them on a parchment-lined cookie sheet. Bake in the preheated oven at 400 degrees F approximately 15 minutes or until they are golden and crisp.

Notes:

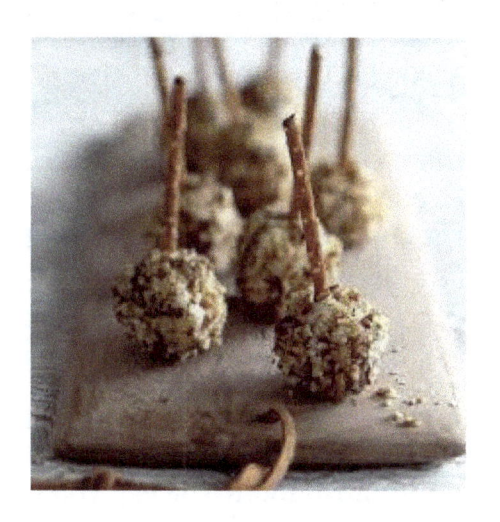

30. Alfredo Cheese Dip

INGREDIENTS (12 servings)

2 tablespoons butter 2 cloves garlic, chopped 1 ½ cups Swiss chard, chopped 1/2 cup Swiss cheese, grated 1 ½ cups Ricotta cheese, softened 1/2 cup Prosciutto, roughly chopped 6 ounces double cream 2 egg yolks Salt and pepper, to taste

DIRECTIONS (30 minutes)

Strat by preheating your oven to 355 degrees F. In a saucepan, melt the butter over medium-low heat. Cook the cream, salt and pepper for about 3 minutes. Add in the egg yolks and continue to cook for 4 to 5 minutes more, stirring continuously. Spoon the mixture into a baking dish. Add in the remaining ingredients and stir to combine. Bake in the preheated oven for 18 to 20 minutes.Enjoy!

Notes:

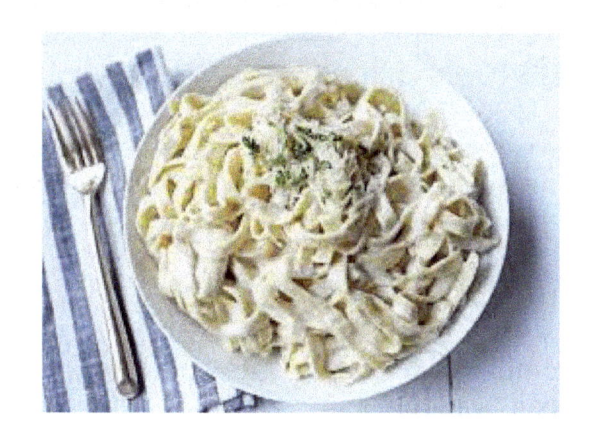

31. Genovese Salami and Egg Fat Bombs

INGREDIENTS (6 servings)

6 ounces Genovese salami, chopped 2 hard-boiled eggs, chopped 1 ½ tablespoons fresh cilantro, chopped 6 ounces cream cheese Salt and pepper, to taste

DIRECTIONS (5 minutes)

Thoroughly combine all ingredients until well incorporated. Shape into 12 balls.Enjoy!

Notes:

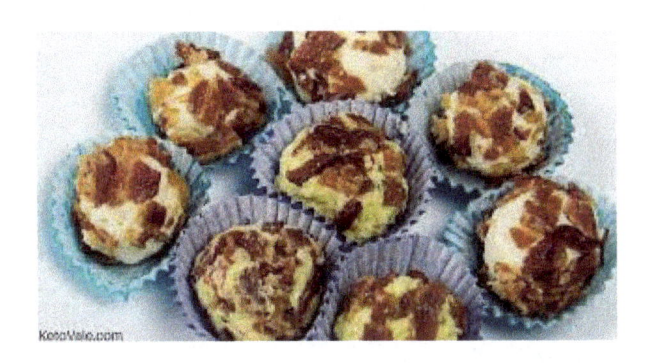

32. Asparagus & Tarragon Flan

INGREDIENTS (4 servings)

16 asparagus, stems trimmed ½ cup whipping cream 1 cup almond milk 2 eggs + 2 egg yolks, beaten in a bowl 2 tbsp fresh tarragon, chopped Salt and black pepper to taste 2 tbsp Parmesan cheese, grated 2 tbsp butter, melted 1 tbsp butter, softened

DIRECTIONS (65 minutes)

Cover the asparagus with salted water and bring them to boil over medium heat for 6 minutes. Drain the asparagus, cut their tips, and reserve for garnishing. Chop the remaining asparagus into small pieces. In a blender, add chopped asparagus, whipping cream, almond milk, tarragon, salt, pepper, and Parmesan cheese. Process until smooth. Pour the mixture through a sieve into a bowl and whisk in the eggs. Preheat oven to 350°F. Grease 4 ramekins with softened butter and share the asparagus mixture among the ramekins. Pour the melted butter over each mixture and top with 2-3 asparagus tips. Pour 3 cups water into a baking dish, place in the ramekins, and insert in the oven. Bake for 45 minutes until their middle parts are no longer watery. Remove the ramekins and let cool. Garnish the flan with the asparagus tips and serve with chilled white wine.

Notes:

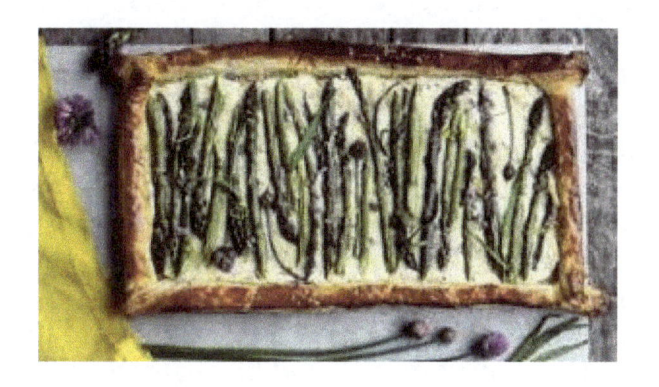

33. Tofu Sandwich with Cabbage Slaw

INGREDIENTS (4 servings)

½ lb firm tofu, sliced 4 zero carb buns 1 tbsp olive oil Marinade Salt and black pepper to taste 2 tsp allspice 1 tbsp erythritol 2 tsp chopped thyme 1 habanero pepper, minced 3 green onions, thinly sliced 2 cloves garlic ¼ cup olive oil Slaw ½ small cabbage, shredded 1 carrot, grated ½ red onion, grated ½ tsp swerve sugar 2 tbsp white vinegar 1 tsp Italian seasoning ¼ cup olive oil 1 tsp Dijon mustard Salt and black pepper to taste

DIRECTIONS (10 minutes)

In a food processor, make the marinade by blending the allspice, salt, black pepper, erythritol, thyme, habanero, green onions, garlic, and olive oil, for a minute. Pour the mixture into a bowl and put in the tofu. Toss to coat. Place in the fridge to marinate for 4 hours. In a large bowl, combine the white vinegar, swerve sugar, olive oil, mustard, Italian seasoning, salt, and pepper. Stir in the cabbage, carrot, and onion and place it in the refrigerator to chill. Heat 1 teaspoon of oil in a skillet over medium heat, remove the tofu from the marinade, and cook it in the oil to brown on both sides for 6 minutes in total. Remove onto a plate after and toast the buns in the skillet. In the buns, add the tofu and top with the slaw. Close the bread and serve with a sweet chili sauce.

Notes:

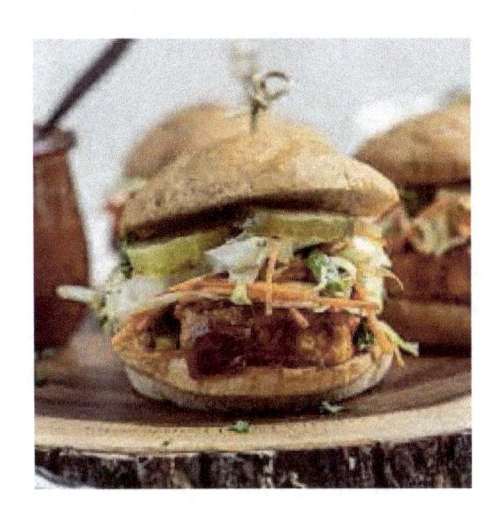

34. Lemon Cauliflower "Couscous" with Halloumi

INGREDIENTS (4 servings)

4 oz halloumi, sliced 2 tbsp olive oil 1 cauliflower head, cut into florets ¼ cup chopped cilantro ¼ cup chopped parsley ¼ cup chopped mint ½ lemon juiced Salt and black pepper to taste 1 avocado, sliced to garnish

DIRECTIONS (5 minutes)

Warm the olive oil in a skillet over medium heat. Add the halloumi and fry for 2 minutes on each side until golden brown; set aside. Pour the cauli florets in a food processor and pulse until it crumbles and resembles couscous. Transfer to a bowl and steam in the microwave for 2 minutes. Remove the bowl from the microwave and let the cauli cool. Stir in cilantro, parsley, mint, lemon juice, salt, and pepper. Top couscous with avocado slices and serve with grilled halloumi and vegetable sauce.

Notes:

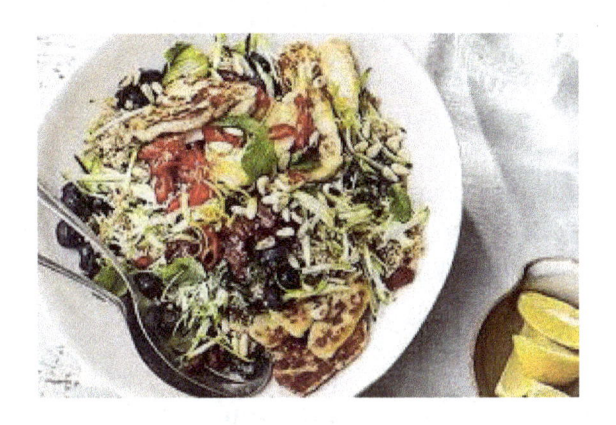

35. Zucchini Lasagna with Ricotta & Spinach

INGREDIENTS (4 servings)

2 zucchinis, sliced Salt and black pepper to taste 2 cups ricotta cheese 2 cups shredded mozzarella cheese 3 cups tomato sauce 1 cup baby spinach Preheat oven to 370°F.

DIRECTIONS (50 minutes)

Put the zucchini slices in a colander and sprinkle with salt. Let sit and drain liquid for 5 minutes and pat dry with paper towels. Mix the ricotta cheese, mozzarella cheese, salt, and black pepper to evenly combine and spread ¼ cup of the mixture in the bottom of the baking dish. Layer ⅓ of the zucchini slices on top, spread 1 cup of tomato sauce over, and scatter a ⅓ cup of spinach on top. Repeat the layering process two more times to exhaust the ingredients while finally making sure to layer with the last ¼ cup of cheese mixture. Grease one end of foil with cooking spray and cover the baking dish with the foil. Bake for 35 minutes, remove foil, and bake further for 5 to 10 minutes or until the cheese has a nice golden brown color. Remove the dish, sit for 5 minutes, make slices of the lasagna, and serve warm.

Notes:

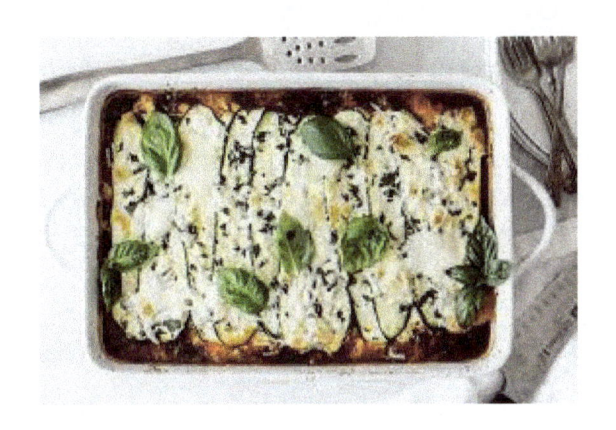

36. Creamy Vegetable Stew

INGREDIENTS (4 servings)

2 tbsp ghee 1 tbsp onion-garlic puree 2 medium carrots, chopped 1 head cauliflower, cut into florets 2 cups green beans, halved Salt and black pepper to taste 1 cup water 1 ½ cups heavy cream

DIRECTIONS (25 minutes)

Melt the ghee in a saucepan over medium heat and sauté onion-garlic puree to be fragrant, 2 minutes. Stir in carrots, cauliflower, and green beans for 5 minutes. Season with salt and black pepper. Pour in the water, stir again, and cook on low heat for 15 minutes. Mix in the heavy cream to be incorporated and turn the heat off. Serve the stew with almond flour bread

Notes:

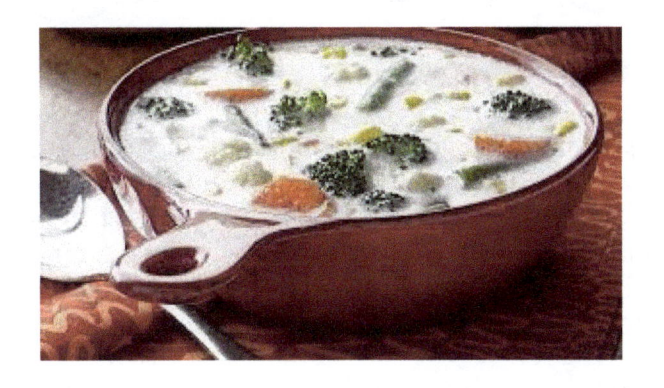

37. Salami & Prawn Pizza

INGREDIENTS (6 servings)

1 low carb pizza crust (see "Homemade Pizza Crust") 1 cup sugar-free pizza sauce 2 ¼ cups mozzarella cheese, grated 4 oz Hot Salami, thinly sliced 3 tomatoes, thinly sliced 16 prawns, deveined and halved 2 cloves garlic, finely sliced 2 cups baby arugula 2 tbsp toasted pine nuts 1 tbsp olive oil Salt and black pepper to taste 10 basil leaves Preheat oven to 450°F.

DIRECTIONS (35 minutes)

With the pizza bread on the pizza pan, spread the pizza sauce on it and sprinkle with half of the mozzarella cheese. Top with the salami, tomatoes, prawns, and garlic, then sprinkle the remaining cheese over it. Place the pizza in the oven to bake for 15 minutes. Once the cheese has melted, top with the basil leaves. In a bowl, toss the arugula and pine nuts with olive oil and adjust its seasoning to taste. Section the pizza with a slicer and serve with the arugula mixture.

Notes:

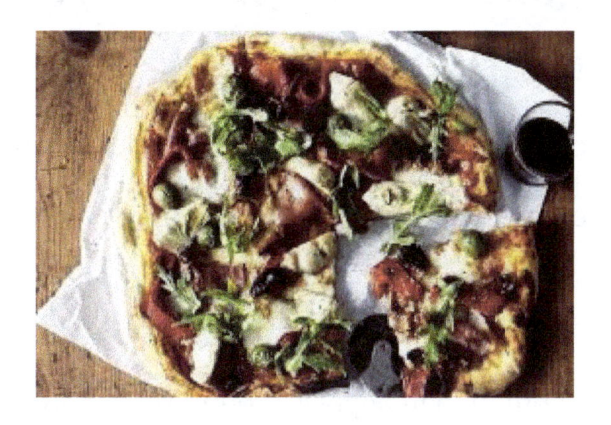

38. Pork & Vegetable Tart

INGREDIENTS (6 servings)

2 lb ground pork 1 onion, chopped 1 bell pepper, chopped Salt and black pepper to taste 2 zucchinis, sliced 2 tomatoes, sliced ¼ cup whipping cream 8 eggs ½ cup Monterey Jack cheese, grated Preheat oven to 360°F.

DIRECTIONS (45 minutes)

In a bowl, mix onion, bell pepper, ground pork, pepper, and salt. Layer the mixture on a greased baking dish. Spread zucchini slices on top, followed by tomato slices. Bake for 30 minutes. In a separate bowl, combine cheese, eggs, and whipping cream. Top the tart with the creamy mixture and bake for 10 minutes until the edges and top become brown. Let cool slightly, slice, and serve.

Notes:

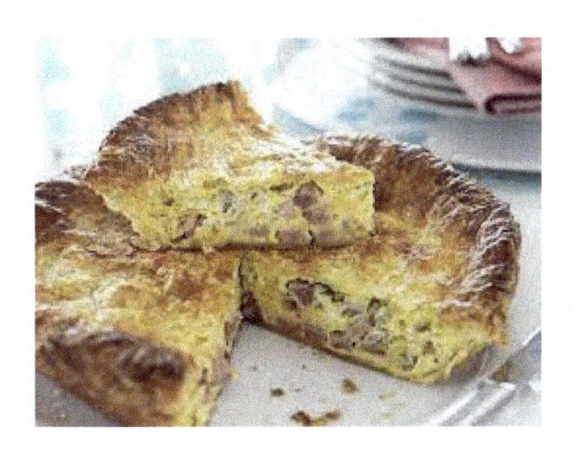

39. Ham & Egg Salad

INGREDIENTS (4 servings)

4 eggs 1 cup mayonnaise 1 green onion, sliced diagonally ½ tsp mustard 1 tsp lime juice Salt and black pepper to taste 1 small lettuce, torn ½ cup ham, chopped

DIRECTIONS (20 minutes)

Boil the eggs in salted water for 10 minutes. Remove and run under cold water. Peel and chop them. Remove to a mixing bowl together with the mayonnaise, mustard, black pepper, ham, lime juice, and salt. Lay on a bed of lettuce. Scatter the green onion over and serve.

Notes:

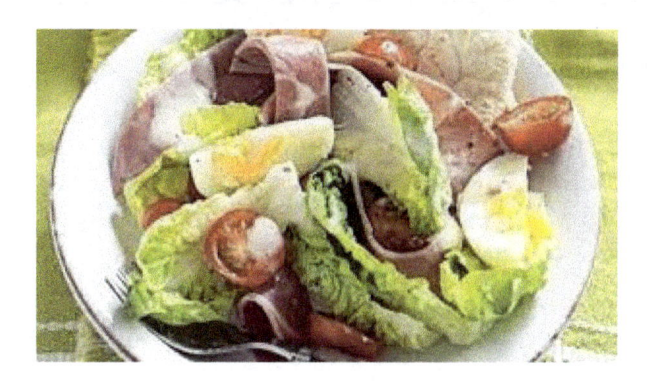

40. Greek Yogurt & Cheese Alfredo Sauce

INGREDIENTS (12 servings)

2 tbsp butter 6 oz heavy cream Salt and black pepper to taste 2 cloves garlic, chopped ¾ cup sour cream ½ cup Gruyere cheese, grated 1 cup goat cheese ½ cup cooked bacon, chopped 1 cup Greek yogurt

DIRECTIONS (10 minutes)

Set a pan over medium heat and warm butter. Stir in heavy cream and cook for 2-3 minutes. Sprinkle with black pepper and salt; mix in the Greek yogurt and cook for 2 minutes. Stir in the remaining ingredients to mix well until smooth. Serve.

Notes:

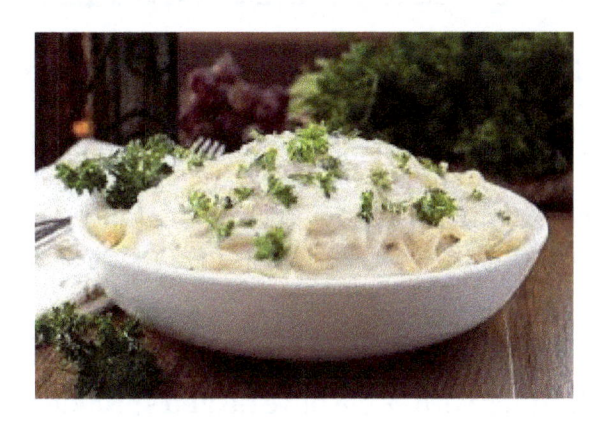

41. Broccoli Rabe Pizza with Parmesan

INGREDIENTS (2 servings)

1 cauliflower pizza crust 2 tbsp olive oil 2 parsnips, chopped Salt and black pepper to taste 2 cups broccoli rabe 2 hard-boiled eggs, chopped ½ cup largely diced bacon 1 cup grated Parmesan cheese 2 tbsp chopped basil leaves Preheat oven to 400°F.

DIRECTIONS (40 minutes)

Drizzle the parsnips with some olive oil and sprinkle with salt and pepper. Place on a baking sheet. Bake for 20 minutes; set aside. Toss the broccoli rabe with 2 tablespoons of olive oil in a bowl, season with salt and pepper, and drain any liquid from the bowl. Bake the crust for 7 minutes. Let cool for a few minutes and brush with the remaining olive oil. Scatter the parsnips all over, top with the broccoli rabe, bacon, and eggs, and sprinkle with Parmesan cheese. Bake for 6-8 minutes until the cheese is melted. Garnish with basil and section with a pizza cutter. Serve with sundried tomato salad.

Notes:

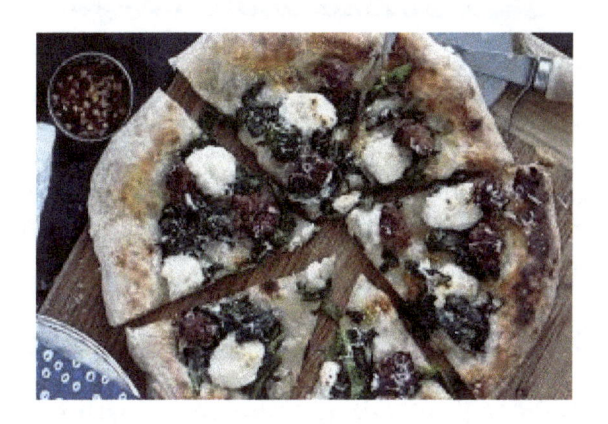

42. Chorizo Scotch Eggs

INGREDIENTS (4 servings)

4 whole eggs 1 egg, beaten ½ cup pork rinds, crushed 1 lb chorizo sausages, skinless ¼ cup Grana Padano cheese, grated 1 garlic clove, minced ¼ tsp onion powder ¼ tsp chili pepper Salt and black pepper to taste

DIRECTIONS (35 minutes)

Cook the eggs in boiling salted water over medium heat for 10 minutes. Rinse under running water and remove the shell; reserve. Preheat oven to 370°F. In a mixing dish, mix the other ingredients, except for the beaten egg and pork rinds. Take a handful of the mixture and wrap around each of the boiled eggs. With fingers, mold the mixture until sealed to form balls. Dip the balls in the beaten eggs, coat with rinds, and place in a greased baking dish. Bake for 25 minutes, until golden brown and crisp. Serve chilled.

Notes:

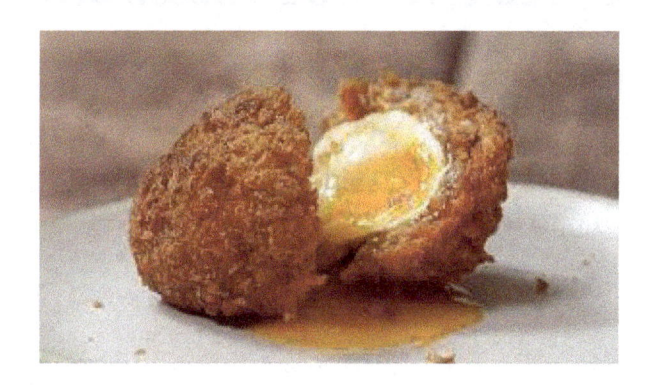

43. Mediterranean Cheese Balls

INGREDIENTS (6 servings)

4 oz prosciutto, chopped 4 oz goat cheese, crumbled ½ cup aioli ½ cup black olives, chopped ½ tsp red pepper flakes 2 tbsp fresh basil, finely chopped

DIRECTIONS (5 minutes)

In a bowl, mix aioli, prosciutto, goat cheese, red pepper flakes, and black olives. Form 10 balls from the mixture. Roll them in the basil. Arrange on a serving platter and serve immediately.

Notes:

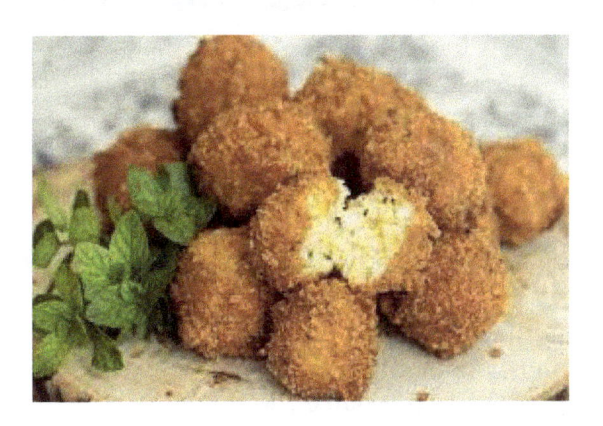

44. Ham & Egg Mug Cups

INGREDIENTS (2 servings)

4 eggs 4 tbsp coconut milk ¼ cup ham, cubed ½ tsp chili pepper Salt and black pepper to taste 2 tbsp chives, chopped

DIRECTIONS (5 minutes)

Mix all ingredients, excluding chives. Divide the egg mixture into 2 greased microwave-safe cups. Microwave for 1 minute. Decorate with chives before serving.

Notes:

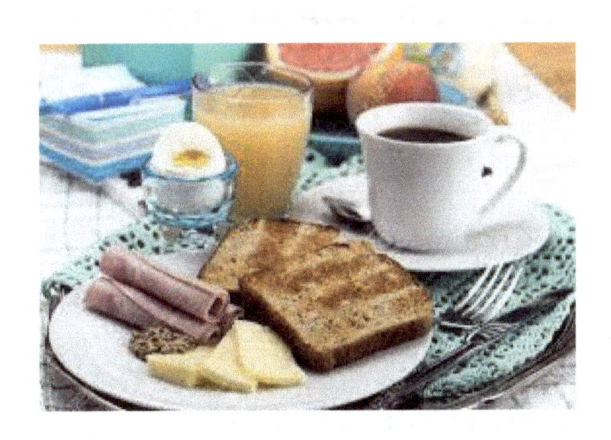

45. Cauliflower & Gouda Cheese Casserole

INGREDIENTS (4 servings)

2 heads cauliflower, cut into florets 2 tbsp olive oil 2 tbsp butter, melted 1 white onion, chopped Salt and black pepper to taste ¼ almond milk ½ cup almond flour 1 ½ cups gouda cheese, grated Preheat oven to 350°F.

DIRECTIONS (25 minutes)

Put the cauli florets in a large microwave-safe bowl. Sprinkle with a bit of water, and steam in the microwave for 4 to 5 minutes. Warm the olive oil in a saucepan over medium heat and sauté the onion for 3 minutes. Add the cauliflower, season with salt and pepper, and mix in almond milk. Simmer for 3 minutes. Mix the melted butter with almond flour. Stir into the cauliflower as well as half of the cheese. Sprinkle the top with the remaining cheese and bake for 10 minutes until the cheese has melted and golden brown on the top. Plate the bake and serve with salad.

Notes:

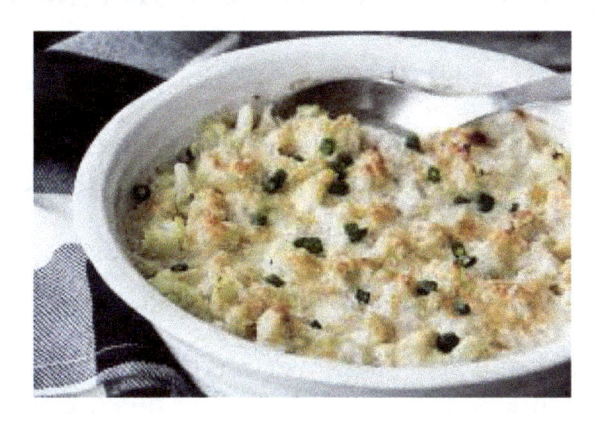

46. Cremini Mushroom Stroganoff

INGREDIENTS (4 servings)

3 tbsp butter 1 white onion, chopped 4 cups cremini mushrooms, cubed ½ cup heavy cream ½ cup Parmesan cheese, grated 1 ½ tbsp dried mixed herbs

DIRECTIONS (25 minutes)

Melt the butter in a saucepan over medium heat and sauté the onion for 3 minutes until soft. Stir in the mushrooms and cook until tender, about 5 minutes. Add 2 cups water and bring to boil. Cook for 10-15 minutes until the water reduces slightly. Pour in the heavy cream and Parmesan cheese. Stir to melt the cheese. Mix in the dried herbs and season. Simmer for 5 minutes. Serve warm.

Notes:

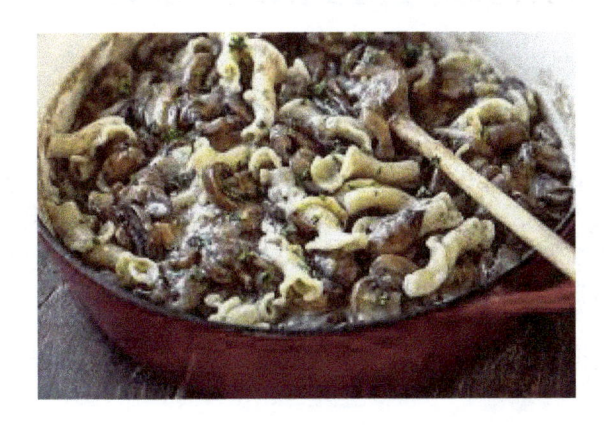

47. Sriracha Tofu with Yogurt Sauce

INGREDIENTS (4 servings)

12 oz tofu, pressed and sliced 1 cup green onions, chopped 1 garlic clove, minced 2 tbsp vinegar 1 tbsp sriracha sauce 2 tbsp olive oil Yogurt sauce 2 cloves garlic, pressed 2 tbsp fresh lemon juice Salt and black pepper to taste 1 tsp fresh dill weed 1 cup Greek yogurt 1 cucumber, shredded

DIRECTIONS (40 minutes)

Put tofu slices, garlic, sriracha sauce, vinegar, and green onions in a bowl. Allow to settle for 30 minutes. Set a nonstick skillet to medium heat and add oil to warm. Cook tofu for 5 minutes until golden brown. For the preparation of the sauce: In a bowl, mix garlic, salt, yogurt, black pepper, lemon juice, and dill. Add in shredded cucumber as you stir to combine. Serve the tofu with a dollop of yogurt sauce.

Notes:

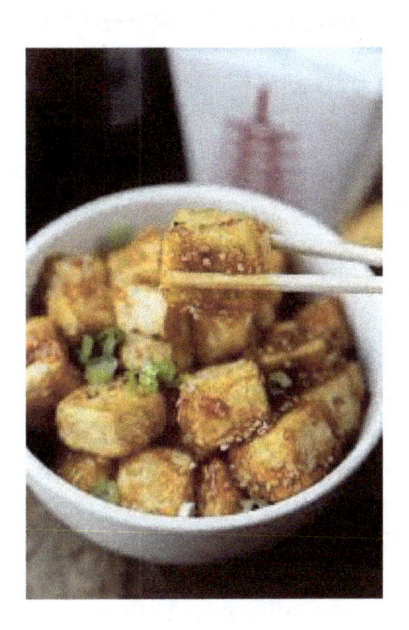

48. Wild Mushroom & Asparagus Stew

INGREDIENTS (4 servings)

2 tbsp olive oil 1 onion, chopped 2 garlic cloves, pressed 1 celery stalk, chopped 2 carrots, chopped 1 cup wild mushrooms, sliced 2 tbsp dry white wine 2 rosemary sprigs, chopped 1 thyme sprig, chopped 2 cups vegetable stock ½ tsp chili pepper 1 tsp smoked paprika 2 tomatoes, chopped 1 tbsp flaxseed meal

DIRECTIONS (25 minutes)

Warm the olive oil in a pot over medium heat. Add in onions and cook until tender, about 3 minutes. Place in carrots, celery, and garlic and cook until soft for 4 more minutes. Add in mushrooms and cook until the liquid evaporates; set aside. Stir in wine to deglaze the pot's bottom. Place in thyme and rosemary. Pour in tomatoes, vegetable stock, paprika, and chili pepper, add in reserved vegetables, and bring to a boil. Reduce the heat to low and let the mixture to simmer for 15 minutes. Stir in flaxseed meal to thicken the stew, about 2-3 minutes. Spoon into individual bowls and serve warm.

Notes:

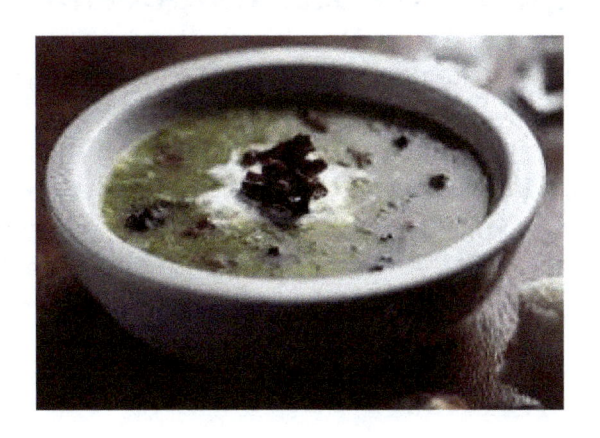

49. Keto Pizza Margherita

INGREDIENTS (2 servings)

Crust 6 oz mozzarella cheese, grated 2 tbsp cream cheese, softened 2 tbsp Parmesan cheese, grated 1 tsp dried oregano ½ cup almond flour 2 tbsp psyllium husk Topping 4 oz cheddar cheese, grated ¼ cup marinara sauce 1 bell pepper, sliced 1 tomato, sliced 2 tbsp fresh basil, chopped Preheat oven to 400°F.

DIRECTIONS (25 minutes)

Melt the mozzarella cheese in a microwave. Combine the remaining crust ingredients in a large bowl and add the mozzarella cheese. Mix with your hands to combine. Divide the dough in two. Roll out the two crusts in circles and place on a lined baking sheet. Bake for 10 minutes. Remove and spread the marinara sauce evenly. Top with cheddar cheese, bell pepper, and tomato slices. Return to the oven and bake for 10 more minutes. Serve sliced sprinkled with basil.

Notes:

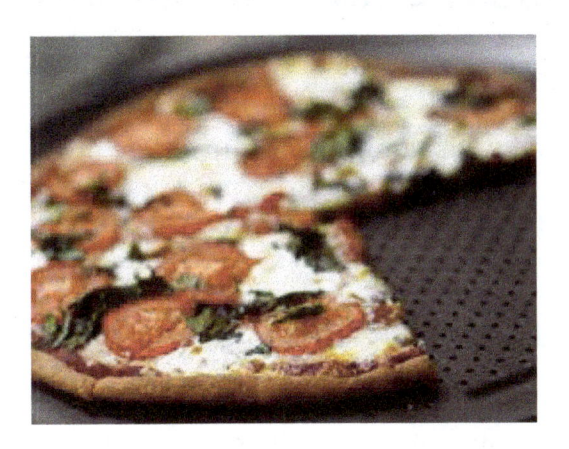

50. Cauliflower Risotto with Mushrooms

INGREDIENTS (4 servings)

2 shallots, diced 2 tbsp olive oil ¼ cup veggie broth ⅓ cup Parmesan cheese, shredded 2 tbsp butter 3 tbsp chives, chopped 1 lb mushrooms, sliced 4 cups cauliflower rice Salt and black pepper to taste

DIRECTIONS (15 minutes)

Heat olive oil in a saucepan over medium heat. Add the mushrooms and shallots and cook for 5 minutes until tender. Set aside. Add in the cauliflower, broth, salt, and pepper and cook until the liquid is absorbed, about 4-5 minutes. Stir in butter and Parmesan cheese until the cheese is melted. Serve warm.

Notes:

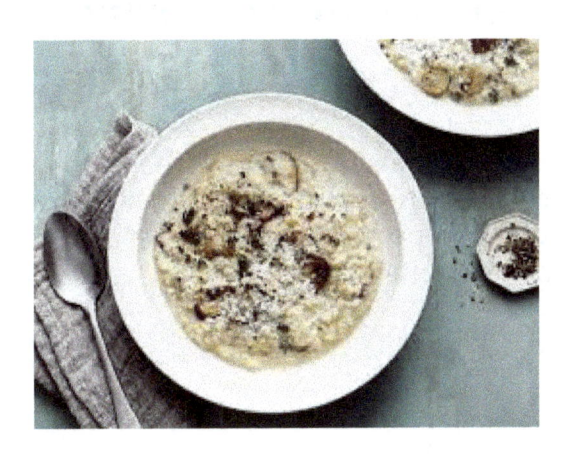

51. Walnut Tofu Sauté

INGREDIENTS (4 servings)

1 tbsp olive oil 1 (8 oz) block firm tofu, cubed 1 tbsp tomato paste 1 garlic clove, minced 1 onion, chopped 1 tbsp balsamic vinegar Salt and black pepper to taste ½ tsp mixed dried herbs 1 cup chopped raw walnuts

DIRECTIONS (15 minutes)

Heat the oil in a skillet over medium heat and cook the tofu for 3 minutes until brown. Stir in the garlic, onion, tomato paste, and vinegar and cook for 4 minutes. Season with salt and pepper. Add in the herbs and walnuts. Stir and cook on low heat for 3 minutes. Spoon on plates and serve warm.

Notes:

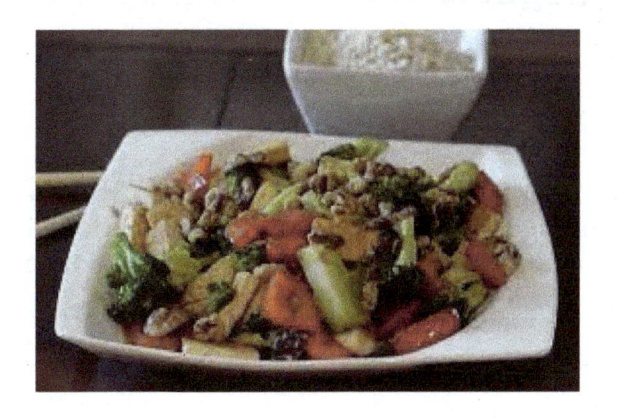

52. Spaghetti Squash with Eggplant & Parmesan

INGREDIENTS (4 servings)

2 tbsp butter 1 cup cherry tomatoes 1 eggplant, cubed ¼ cup Parmesan cheese, shredded 3 tbsp scallions, chopped 1 cup snap peas 1 tsp lemon zest 2 cups spaghetti squash, cooked Salt and black pepper to taste

DIRECTIONS (15 minutes)

Melt butter in a saucepan and cook eggplant for 5 minutes until tender. Add in the tomatoes and peas and cook for 5 minutes. Stir in the zest, scallions, salt, and pepper. Remove the pan from heat. Stir in spaghetti squash and Parmesan cheese and serve.

Notes:

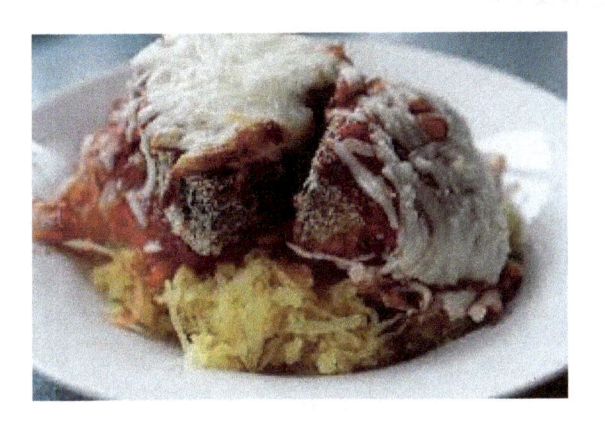

53. Fried Tofu with Mushrooms

INGREDIENTS (2 servings)

12 oz extra-firm tofu, cubed 1 ½ tbsp flaxseed meal Salt and black pepper to taste 1 tsp garlic clove, minced ½ tsp paprika 1 tsp onion powder 2 tbsp olive oil 1 cup mushrooms, sliced 1 jalapeño pepper, deveined, sliced

DIRECTIONS (40 minutes)

In a bowl, add onion powder, tofu, salt, paprika, black pepper, jalapeño pepper, flaxseed, and garlic. Toss the mixture to coat and allow to marinate for 30 minutes. Warm the olive oil in a pan over medium heat. Cook mushrooms for 5 minutes until tender, stirring continuously. Add in the tofu mixture and stir. Cook for 4-5 more minutes. Divide between plates and serve warm.

Notes:

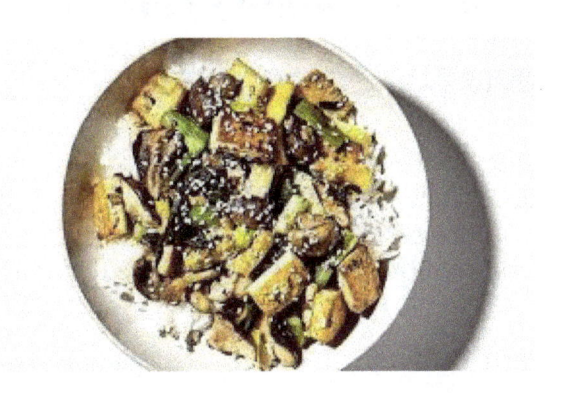

54. Vegetable Tempura

INGREDIENTS (4 servings)

½ cup coconut flour + extra for dredging Salt and black pepper to taste 3 egg yolks 2 red bell peppers, cut into strips 1 squash, peeled and cut into strips 1 broccoli, cut into florets 1 cup chilled water 4 tbsp olive oil 4 lemon wedges ½ cup sugar-free soy sauce

DIRECTIONS (20 minutes)

In a deep frying pan, heat the olive oil over medium heat. Beat the eggs lightly with ½ cup of coconut flour and water. The mixture should be lumpy. Dredge the vegetables lightly in some flour, shake off the excess flour, dip it in the batter, and then into the hot oil. Fry in batches for 1 minute each, not more, and remove with a perforated spoon onto a wire rack. Sprinkle with salt and pepper and serve with the lemon wedges and soy sauce.

Notes:

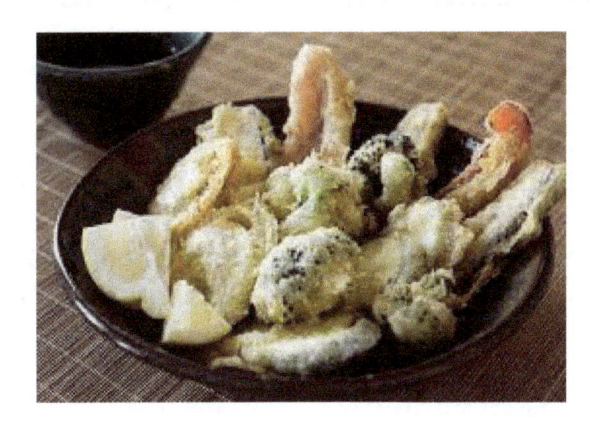

55. Spanish-Style Sausage and Eggs

INGREDIENTS (2 servings)

6 ounces Chorizo sausage, crumbled 4 eggs, whisked 1/2 cup Hojiblanca olives, pitted and sliced 1 teaspoon garlic paste 1 teaspoon ancho chili pepper, deveined and minced 2 tablespoons canola oil 1/2 cup red onions, chopped 2 rosemary sprigs, leaves picked and chopped Salt and black pepper to the taste

DIRECTIONS (20 minutes)

In a frying pan, heat the oil over a moderate flame; cook red onions until just tender and fragrant, about 4 to 5 minutes. Add in the garlic, pepper, salt, black pepper, sausage, and olives; continue to cook, stirring constantly, for 7 to 8 minutes. Stir in the eggs and rosemary leaves; cook for 4 to 5 minutes, lifting and folding the eggs until thickened.Enjoy!

Notes:

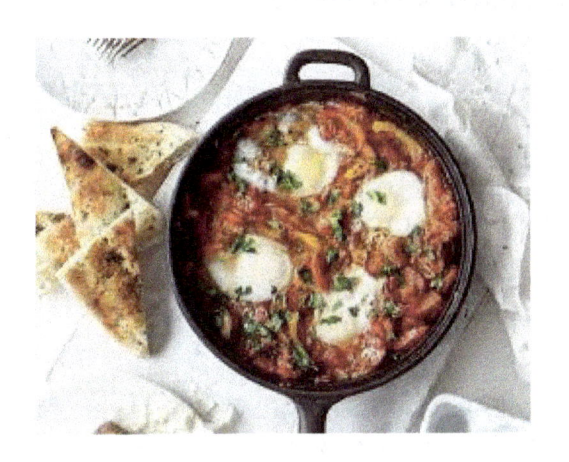

56. Keto Belgian Waffles

INGREDIENTS (6 servings)

3 smoked Belgian sausages, crumbled 1 cup Limburger cheese, shredded 1/2 teaspoon ground cloves 6 eggs 6 tablespoons milk Sea salt and pepper, to taste

DIRECTIONS (30 minutes)

Whisk the eggs with the milk and spices until pale and frothy. Add in the crumbled Belgian sausage and Limburger cheese. Mix until everything is well combined. Brush a waffle iron with a nonstick cooking spray. Pour the batter into waffle iron and cook until golden and cooked through. Repeat until all the batter is used.Enjoy!

Notes:

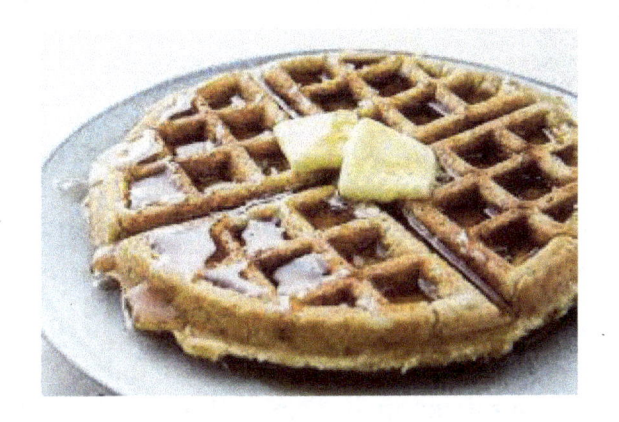

57. Scotch Eggs with Ground Pork

INGREDIENTS (8 servings)

8 eggs 1 ½ pounds ground pork 1/2 cup Romano cheese, freshly grated 1 teaspoon garlic, smashed 1/2 teaspoon onion powder 1/2 teaspoon red pepper flakes, crushed 1 teaspoon Italian seasoning mix

DIRECTIONS (20 minutes)

Place the eggs in a saucepan and cover them with water by 1 inch. Cover and bring water to a boil over high heat. Boil for 6 to 7 minutes over medium-high heat; peel the eggs and rinse them under running water. Thoroughly combine the remaining ingredients. Divide the mixture into 8 pieces; now, using your fingers, shape the meat mixture around the eggs. Bake in the preheated oven at 365 degrees F for 20minutes until golden brown.

Notes:

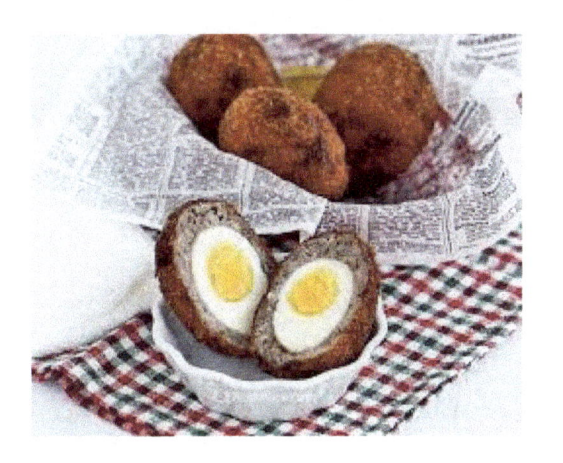

Lightning Source UK Ltd.
Milton Keynes UK
UKHW020923010721
386455UK00005B/76

www.ingramcontent.com/pod-product-compliance
Ingram Content Group UK Ltd.
Pitfield, Milton Keynes, MK11 3LW, UK
UKHW041842141224
452457UK00012B/600